The
Dysthymia
Diaries

True stories of living with dysthymia,
and finding help and hope

Robyn Wheeler

The Dysthymia Diaries

Robyn Wheeler

Disclaimer

Before considering any technique described herein as a form of physical, mental or emotional treatment, the author recommends that you seek the advice of a qualified physician or professional therapist.

BornMad.org
DysthymicDisorder.info
Facebook.com/dysthymicdisorderinformation

ISBN (Print):   978-1-4951-8436-9
ISBN (eBook):   978-1-4951-8437-6

Library of Congress Control Number: 2015920305

First Edition 2016

Dedicated to those who suffer from dysthymic disorder and their families, friends and loved ones. It is for those who have not been diagnosed yet, and are wondering what is wrong with them and why they aren't like everybody else.

The point is dysthymia is a very dysfunctional illness, even relative to acute major depression. Dysthymia is what ruins peoples' lives.

—Dr. Jonathan W. Stewart, Clinical Psychiatry News, Aug. 2010

Many people with dysthymic disorder have no idea they have a mood disorder. They just believe that they are "meant" to be depressed, or that negativity, pessimism, sadness and low energy is just part of their personality.

—Columbia University Medical Center, New York

My life felt like I was eating a bowl of ice cream that had no flavor. Everybody around me seemed capable of enjoying life and I felt like "What is the point?" For too many years, I simply survived and those were the "good" days. When I dipped below a steady flat line, I felt like my soul was being twisted and the pain was forced out like water wrung from a dishtowel.

—Personal letter to Robyn Wheeler from Doreen, San Diego, California

I had gone through my entire life feeling blue, never feeling quite right. I was missing a dimension, a dimension of joy. I don't remember ever experiencing real happiness until I was successfully in recovery from alcoholism. There was rarely any reason for my dark moods, but they transcended everything I did. My internal outlook diminished all peak experiences. I envied other people's rosy perspectives and often wondered how they could feel so good. I felt deprived. I felt like I was missing out on something very basic.

—Vivian Eisenecher, Author of Recovering Me, Discovering Joy: Uplifting Wisdom for Everyday Greatness

Thank you for your website and YouTube videos. I am sitting here crying my eyes out because I feel like I found an answer to my pain and suffering.

—Private letter to Robyn Wheeler from Iceland resident

Dysthymic individuals believe that they must always be good, perfect, right and if they aren't, they're worthless. Yet, please keep in mind that just because neurotic individuals may believe they're inferior and incapable doesn't mean they are. Neurotic persons may wrestle with even the most trivial decisions and perceive them as monumental.

—Dr. Roger Dietro, Psy.D., and
Dr. Harold H. Mosak, Ph.D., ABPP, in
*The Depression Code: Deciphering the
Purposes of Neurotic Depression*

My perspective has a great deal to do with how I feel about things. I can get locked into a negative mindset because of incorrect assumptions. Sometimes just changing my perspective helps me to change my attitude and feelings about a particular thing. When I struggle with emotions and feel besieged with problems, I try to analyze why. This helps me to put things in perspective and, hopefully, react in a healthier way.

—Jenny Hess, Author of *In His Hands: A Mother's Journey
through Grief of Sudden Loss*

Do you feel like Eeyore?

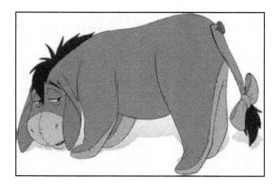

Eeyore: the old grey donkey in Disney's *Winnie the Pooh*. He generally feels pessimistic, complaining, gloomy, anhedonic and depressed. Some who suffer from dysthymic disorder say they identify with Eeyore. If you can identify with Eeyore, you are not alone.

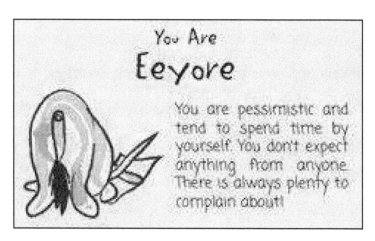

You Are

Eeyore

You are pessimistic and tend to spend time by yourself. You don't expect anything from anyone. There is always plenty to complain about!

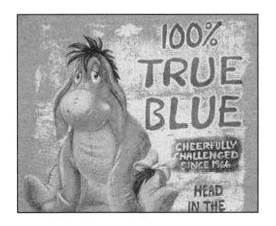

Famous Eeyore Quotes

I'd look on the bright side, if I could find it.

Could be worse. Not sure how, but it could be.

Keep calm and gloom on.

Don't pay any attention to me. Nobody ever does.

For some reason, I'm always getting forgotten.

I never get up my hopes, so I never get let down.

The sky has finally fallen. I always knew it would.

I was so upset, I forgot to be happy.

Contents

Introduction

Dysthymic disorder (now called *persistent depressive disorder* by the *Diagnostic Statistical Manual V*) affects 3 to 6 percent of the population, which is a greater percentage than bipolar disorder and schizophrenia combined. Yet, a larger number of people are more aware of and familiar with the symptoms of bipolar and schizophrenia than they are with dysthymia.

Dysthymia also causes more disability than major depression. According to *Clinical Psychiatry*, Aug. 2010, Dr. Jonathan W. Stewart found dysthymia sufferers topped disability lists even above those with major depression.

In a study of 712 acute major depressive patients, 42,052 of the general population and 328 with dysthymic disorder, here are the results:

- Full-time employment was reported by 36 percent of those with dysthymia, 44 percent by those with major depression and 52 percent of the general population.

- Those accomplishing less due to emotional problems were 13 percent of dysthymics, 8 percent of those with major depression and 3 percent of the general population.

- Those reporting emotional problems interfering with work were 7 percent of dysthymics and those with major depression and 3 percent of the general population.

- Social Security disability was reported by 14 percent of the dysthymic group, 5 percent of those with major depression and 3 percent of the general population.
- Medicaid insurance was reported by 20 percent of the dysthymic group, 13 percent of the major depression group and 6 percent of the general population.

In my view, dysthymia is more than just the "mild" form of depression reported by many psychiatrists. However, its symptoms are considered mild by psychiatrists when compared to bipolar and schizophrenia. For those who suffer from it, dysthymia is far from mild, which is one of the reasons I put together *The Dysthymia Diaries*.

I was diagnosed with dysthymia in 2010 and desperately wanted to connect with someone else who suffered from it. I attempted to find a book written by someone with dysthymic disorder but was unable to track one down. After I wrote my story, *Born Mad*, I began to invite others with dysthymic disorder to write their story as well.

Dysthymic disorder is similar to other spectrum disorders in that everyone who suffers from the mild form of depression may not experience the same symptoms or in the same intensity.

Dysthymic disorder can be insidious and sneaky. Most people who suffer from it, at one point in their lives, did not believe they had any kind of disorder. But dysthymia is there, waiting to attack. Dysthymia will be revealed in your life based on how you respond to circumstances. Those with dysthymic disorder may have few or no coping skills, so that, in challenging times, it rears its ugly head. Although I was first diagnosed with dysthymic disorder at age 44, I will say I've had the disorder my entire life. It was always there. I just didn't realize I was always mildly depressed until I became suicidal and wondered how I went from one extreme to another so quickly. I may have felt "normal" and not depressed, but my happiness baseline was much lower than others'. When I experienced challenging times, I slid downhill fast and hard because my depression was always there. It kicked me in the butt in what seemed like a very short time, but it had been taking its toll all along. It took dire circumstances to reveal my dysthymic state of mind.

According to www.medscape.com, Dysthymia can be divided into two subtypes: *anxious* and *anergic*. Those with anxious dysthymia have pronounced symptoms of low self-esteem, undirected restlessness, and interpersonal rejection sensitivity. They are also characterized as help-seeking, more likely to make lower-lethality suicide attempts and have a better response to selective serotonin reuptake inhibitors (SSRIs). When attempting to self-medicate, substances of choice for this type include benzodiazepines, alcohol, marijuana, opiates and possibly food.

Anergic (without anxiety) dysthymics have low energy, hypersomnia (sleeping too much) and the inability to experience pleasure while participating in normally pleasurable acts (anhedonia). Anergic dysthymics are less likely to be impulsive, have a decreased appetite and a decreased interest in engaging in sexual relations. They also are less likely to ask for help and tend to make more serious, fatal suicide attempts.

These dysthymia sufferers may have a better response to treatment with agents that increase norepinephrine or dopamine.

I experience chronic anger with my dysthymia. Little things can upset me and I can stay mad for days, weeks or even months. I also experience low self-esteem, fatigue, poor concentration and difficulty making decisions.

Others may experience anger or the other symptoms I do in less intensity and frequency or not at all. Still others may have intense feelings of doom, hopeless or guilt. Some may lack motivation, concentration and/or self-esteem, while others may feel hopeless, worthless, empty, and irritable or suffer from chronic anxiety.

Regardless of the symptoms a person experiences, it does not take away from the fact that dysthymia is real and can lead to worsening of symptoms. Dysthymia affects not only the dysthymic individual but their family, friends, coworkers and many others as well.

While reading the stories in Part 1, please keep in mind a few points.

First, the personal stories in this book range in content because they are written by different people of various ages and geographical locations. Some stories give the reader a sense of hope, whereas others may not, and still other readers may find the same story depressing. These stories were not written to elicit a particular feeling or thought from the reader; instead, they were written to illustrate how varied and complex this disorder can be.

Second, some of these stories contain swearing, foul language and adult content. Some write about past abuse, unhappy childhoods and family life and drug addiction or substance abuse.

These stories were written to give readers a greater sense of what those who have dysthymic disorder struggle with on a daily basis. They were not written to cause the reader grief, sadness or depression. Those who contributed personal stories to this book did so of their own free will, as a means to educate and inform those with dysthymic disorder (diagnosed or undiagnosed) and those who do not suffer from it but may have friends or relatives who do.

As a writer and dysthymia sufferer, I wish I had more stories to share with you. I did, in fact, have several more, but many changed their minds about contributing and some contacted me saying they just couldn't bring themselves to write their stories down.

It is something that is difficult to speak about, and many who suffer from low self-esteem simply cannot bring themselves to write about all the difficulties they have experienced for fear of the shame, guilt and deepening depression they will feel.

Thankfully, the writers who contributed to this book felt their story was worth telling in order to help others.

Part 1:

Personal Stories

Dysthymia in the African-American Community

I was often told I should have nothing to be depressed about because, historically speaking, life has always been difficult for people of color. Medical care, particularly psychiatric care, was very scarce for African-Americans. Resources for diagnosing and treating mental illness were virtually non-existent when I was growing up, and the cost was so astronomical that attempting to seek help was discouraging.

I grew up in the 1970–80s watching *Charlie's Angels* and *Miami Vice*, and listening to Boy George and New Edition. I was the youngest of five, three boys and two girls. My father died when I was just 19 months old, so I had no positive male role model in my life. I was a chubby, quiet, smart kid. I could read and write by the time I was 3 years old.

My earliest memories are of being bullied and picked on by my classmates in school. My mom often worked six days a week and was so weary. I felt bad coming home "tattling" about my school experiences; after all, what could she do to solve them? My siblings didn't give me a lot of sympathy, so I stopped sharing things with them, too. I recall going through most of the second and third grade without talking because no one would talk to me. My first suicide attempt was at age 11. I told a teacher I was lonely walking around the playground by myself, and I asked if she would ask someone to play with me. She said, "I don't get paid enough to find friends for you, so go away and stop bothering people." That afternoon I went home and took a rusty X-ACTO® knife to my wrist. The edge was so jagged and dull; I only succeeded in making an ugly gash. I patched it up with several BAND-AIDs® and told my mother I skinned it rough-housing with the dog.

I think of how early on in my life I knew I was depressed, which was probably around 7 or 8 years of age. I didn't know to give it a specific name; I only knew I was sad all the time. I remember going outside on my back porch or locking myself in the bathroom to cry after I got home from school. I rarely looked forward to birthdays or holidays because of the over-whelming feelings of sadness. Not only because there weren't any gifts, but sometimes I had been forgotten altogether. On my mom's side of the family, I was the youngest of 13 cousins. Usually when the teens got together, I had to stay home, so I just sat in my bedroom closet and read to myself. On my dad's side, I was shunned for not being as pretty as the other girls, so I never went around them at all. It hurt when I would hear other kids talking about going to their grandparent's homes, vacations or family reunions. The best words I could use to describe myself are *misfit* or *outcast*; both would suffice.

Today, I receive treatment by taking prescription medication, going to regular counseling sessions and hypno-therapy and striving for a deep understanding and relationship with God.

With regard to people of color, I would say that the resources are definitely more available and accessible than when I was younger. Insurance can cover treatments and medications, and many schools have counselors on staff who are trained in recognizing depressive symptoms in children. I believe the stigma of receiving treatment for a mental or emo-tional disorder continues to carry judgment and criticism among people of color, especially African-Americans. It is seen as a matter of being weak, or looking for pity, rather than a legitimate illness as with cancer or a physical abnormality.

I would like people to know something before it is too late. It is just as critical for African-Americans to take care of themselves mentally and emotionally as well as physically. I was often chastised and dismissed by people because (as they put it) "life has always been hard for black people." They would say I was just looking for attention or for people to feel sorry for me, but no one did.

I believe this is what led me to choose clinical psychology as my secondary major in college. I wanted to not only put a name to what I was going through, but maybe, in telling my own story of abuse, help someone else. I don't know if I can or ever will consider myself "cured" or that one day I may give up and end my own life. But I didn't go through with it today. And that is what matters right now.

F. Taylor
Texas, USA
Author of *Pieces of Me* poetry
and artwork published 2009

Pieces of Me

I am 45 years old. I don't ever recall a time in my life when I have been happy.

I was the youngest of five children and reared in Fort Worth, Texas. My father died when I was 19 months old, and my mom had to work long hours to support us. Although I was an academically gifted child who excelled in school, I was bullied, beaten and tormented almost every day of my public-school education. I had no friends, and even teachers turned their backs on me when I asked for help.

I rarely spoke of what happened when I got home, because my mother was often stressed out with matters regarding my older siblings, finances, work and other daily matters.

When I was 6 years old, two older male relatives began sexually abusing me, and when I was 8, I was forcibly raped by a young man while staying in the home of an after-school caregiver. The abuse continued until I was almost 10 years old.

I suppose I began using food as comfort because a steady diet of junk food became customary for me. Eventually, I weighed almost 500 pounds (like in the movie *Precious*). In spite of it all, I got a full scholarship to college and minored in Clinical Psychology in an effort to help myself in ways I could otherwise not afford.

Almost everyone who knew my mother would tell her that something was wrong with me, but we simply could not afford the kind of care I needed.

I would go outside to cry, where no one else could see me, and I attempted suicide the first time by cutting my wrists when I was 11 years old.

Two more attempts followed on my 16th birthday and shortly after I graduated from college at 22. I never told anyone what I was going through because it didn't seem to me it would do any good, nor did anyone care. My mother died almost 20 years ago without knowing my story, and my siblings and their children don't understand the long-standing effects of untreated depression. I have given them thousands of dollars which they've never repaid, because I was trying to buy their love. Today, they don't even speak to me.

Not a day goes by when I haven't thought about dying. I spend holidays and birthdays alone; I've never been married; I have no children and only one or two friends.

I am ashamed of my appearance, because since I had gastric bypass surgery to lose weight three years ago, almost all of my hair has fallen out. I have taken various medications for my illness, but they don't seem to do any good after a while or they cause adverse reactions.

If there would be any meaning to my life before it is over, I would wish that I could write a book or speak to people about depression (dysthymia) and why it should be treated as soon as you think something is wrong.

F. Taylor
Texas, USA
Author of *Pieces of Me* poetry
and artwork (2009)

I Exist, I Persist

"I didn't want to write it down. Telling the facts of your life, even at the really low times, like I feel now, can be really demanding of strength and the will to do so. Today is October 4, 2007."

This is the way I began my diary eight years ago. I thought I was chronicling a typical account of a boring 13-year-old black girl's life. I was an only child, pretty and gifted, but all that didn't matter to me. I knew I was depressed, I knew I was suffering, but I didn't know it wasn't just me.

For a long time Dysthymia was just the "Ms. Verbo disease." A code word I made up to describe the combination of irritability, moodiness and self-evasive behavior which controlled my social life. Even then I realized I wasn't supposed to feel lonely around family and friends, or think I wasn't worthy of the happiness that I swore others had amongst themselves. What could have easily been resentment and anger at the lack-luster life I was dealt became sarcasm, self-hate, and eventually numbness.

This was a cycle of self-blame and feelings of unworthiness and as a devout Seventh Day Adventist, I interpreted it as the unworthiness of God's love. The unworthiness justified the feelings of depression in my heart and the inability to change myself permanently. In my most spiritual moments of prayer when I was begging God to fix me, I remember thinking that the Holy Spirit had left my heart as the depression seeped up in its place. I felt I was an unworthy vessel of the lord. I know now, this is furthest from the truth.

At the time I was growing up a conflicted teen like two different people in one body. I was an actress of sorts, because I knew crying and showing my true despair was not acceptable. I also knew having a nihilistic nature would not win me friends or a positive public image. At school, I strived to be the creative, smart, pretty girl, who was just shy. At home, the perfect daughter who didn't give anyone too much trouble and made everyone proud. Despite my acts, I failed miserably at being Ms. Verbo and I hated myself for it.

I hated myself all the way into college and gained 60 pounds because of it. I also lost a loved one and soon after, my high school sweetheart left me for his best friend. It was then, when I was living in the dormitories, after sleeping from 3 a.m. to 7 p.m. for weeks, that I decided I needed help.

When I discovered dysthymia and the "double depression," I was actually genuinely happy for three whole days. It was no longer the "Ms. Verbo disease." It had a name! Therapy began soon after through the counseling program at my university, though it was infrequent and unpredictable. I'd speak to someone for 40 minutes every three weeks or so. I remember going in on a particularly bad day. I was feeling so worthless, impossibly low, and needed help. I wanted to shut off my brain; a recurring thought I was having was "I hate myself, I hate my life, I hate everything."

I came to see my therapist for an emergency check-in, and I'll never forget what she said. She told me that emergency drop-in was for people who were suicidal and needed immediate help. I thought to myself, *So I have to cut myself and bleed open for you to believe I'm worthy of this emergency?* So dysthymia, hating yourself and your life so much for more than 2 years,(in my case 10), isn't enough to warrant an emergency 15-minute session? I was heartbroken. I felt rejected on so many levels. I called my mother, and ranted and cried. It was a life-changing moment for me. It made me question psychological practices and diagnosis. Because anyone who ever experienced what I had gone through would realize there is nothing mild, minor or "less severe" about my depression than being suicidal. I used to envy major depression. I thought, *These people get down for two weeks of hell and then can get back up, while I'm swimming with a cramp in my leg and can't ever stop.*

Eventually it got better for me. I learned better coping mechanisms (from a different psychologist and program). I got regular treatment once a week for three months, tried Wellbutrin for one month but stopped because I realized all the change was coming from me. I didn't need it. I lost weight.

Interestingly enough, I still don't truly know if dysthymia can ever really be separate from me. It's like a growth, really, stuck on my body. Sometimes, I'm ashamed of it, sometimes I'm proud I have thrived despite it. Being a woman of color with a mental illness, more specifically a mood disorder is seemingly a lonely journey. I look for support and understanding but rarely find anyone who has a similar experience I can relate to. I'm hoping my story will be able to help someone who is like me; someone who is young and struggling emotionally, economically and mentally, who exists in a community that does not speak openly about mental illness. I guess I just wanted to say I am here. We exist. We persist.

I was diagnosed with dysthymic disorder in December 2011, my freshman year of college. I've used *https://moodgym.anu .edu.au/login*, which allows me to track how my mood is affecting my actions and thoughts. I also have a great support system of family and a few close friends who have been there for me, especially when college life and financial struggles become more stressful. These people, ironically, are the same people I didn't want to burden with my depression. I am in a good place where I understand that I am not a burden to those who love me.

Ms. Verboten
California, USA

The Zombies Walk Among You

I've lived with dysthymia since I was at least 10. I've been on medication for depression since I was 15, and for dysthymia since I was 27. But except for a two-week period one summer, I'm not sure I've really been alive.

I've always felt a little different, if I can indeed feel. I think I'm missing some essential building block of being human. I am a zombie on a planet desolate of viable brains to eat.

The doctors have their clinical descriptions, but for someone who has lived with dysthymia, it is often difficult to distinguish oneself from the disorder. How much of my mood is me, and how much is the dysthymia?

By definition, dysthymia means "ill humor." To me, dysthymia feels like I'm allergic to happy. Dreams and real life are reversed. I dream in color, I live in gray. I'm on an all-body Novocain® drip.

To quote someone else with the disorder, "Life wanted me dead and I'm still alive." Now doesn't that sound just fun?

Cognitive Behavior Therapy (CBT) was recommended to me. My therapist frequently encouraged me to do things I enjoy. I don't know if she realized that doing almost anything puts me in a state of discomfort and leaves me feeling physically and mentally exhausted. Attempting to act like a normal person puts me in a constant state of discomfort and anxiety. It baffles me that people seem to enjoy my company; it's like they can't see that I'm faulty.

I've been over-medicated and under-medicated. Being on three anti-depressants at once leveled me off so much it was like my mind was in a straightjacket, incapable of making even small adjustments in mood or thought process. Right now, I'm only on one drug, Wellbutrin; and while I have good days, blah days and bad days, at least I feel like I usually have a small say in my moods.

So, how do I deal?

Getting the diagnosis of dysthymia was both worrisome and a relief. My therapist first mentioned it after I snapped at her once too frequently and she asked, "So, are you happy?"

I got annoyed and just blurted out, "This is my normal. I'm not crying all the time, but I'm not bouncing off the walls either. So if that's what 'happy' is, then sure."

Learning that there was actually recognition of something between classic depression and happy was a relief. But learning how little was actually known about it was a big downer; how could I be expected to deal with something so daunting when so little was known about it?

Now I'm focusing on not seeing myself as "a dysthymic person or personality," but as "a person who happens to have dysthymia." I come first. My disorder does not define me.

And since I tend to respond really well to challenges, I challenge myself every day to commit to being a warrior for life and fighting the symptoms. Waking up is always hard because dreaming tends to be so much better than being in the present, but I have hope that one day that will change.

Do I have bad days? Sure. But I have more good days than bad.

While medication has helped, Brazilian Jiu Jitsu has also been hugely instrumental to a more positive state of well-being. It's unique in that it is mentally and physically challenging; you need to live entirely in the present. It requires you to focus on your partner's movements and your own movements, control your breathing and strategize simultaneously while you are in uncomfortable positions. All of this clears my head from the negative thoughts and sets me up for a more optimistic day.

Connecting with support and awareness groups has helped; knowing and relating to others in their trials and triumphs is inspiring.

We're all in this hell of a battle together.

JMS
Colorado, USA

A Game of Ping-Pong

My thoughts felt like they were banging up against my head trying to escape. I imagined them bouncing back and forth off the sides of my skull similar to a ball in a game of Ping-Pong. They slammed against my head faster and faster and harder and harder. It was mentally painful but physically painful, too. I'd never felt anything like it before.

I lay on my bed, crying for hours, wondering what was happening to me. I tried to stop crying as I was making myself sick but unable to stop because of the pain. My husband held me, begging me to keep going, to hang on and wait it out. But I felt hopeless, worthless and exhausted. Convinced life hated me, I begged to die, to be free of the misery, uncertainty and conflict.

Counseling helped temporarily, but every few weeks or so my agony came back. Mediation, anger management and Emotional Freedom Technique (EFT) provided me with fleeting moments of sanity and peace, but still I fell into despair. I was on an emotional rollercoaster with ups and downs, good days, bad days and just plain downright horrible days.

My husband walked on eggshells around me. He knew something was wrong but didn't know how to tell me I needed help or even where to find it.

What causes someone to be angry and depressed when they have a nice home, a great spouse and very few worries or complications in life? I was miserable and didn't know why.

I felt guilty for feeling miserable and angry for no apparent reason. The guilt compounded the misery to an all-time high.

Being in my early 40s, I wondered if I was having a mid-life crisis. Was I bored, burned out, stale? Or was something terribly wrong? My anxiety turned into fear. Fear turned into despair and hopelessness, which then turned into a feeling that I'd be better off dead.

A year later, peace and happiness prevailed. When I begged my counselor for a lobotomy, an exorcism or, at the very least, pot brownies, my counselor instead suggested I visit a psychiatrist.

A week later, I sat in the office waiting for my name to be called, wondering what the doctor would do or say about my condition. An hour later, relief was in sight. The diagnosis of dysthymic disorder was formally on the record and the anti-depressant prescription firmly in my hand.

Dysthymia is a seldom-talked-about, mild form of depression, which, left untreated, is likely to turn into major depression. After researching dysthymic disorder, I realized I'd suffered from this affliction my entire life, since early childhood. Dysthymic disorder affects a greater percentage of the population than schizophrenia and bipolar disorder combined, yet few people are familiar with it.

Today, I feel like a new person. My emotions are under control; I live anger-free more days than not and no longer believe life hates me.

I know I am loved by my family, friends and God, and that life is a journey. My life has already been planned and set into motion, and it is up to me to make my life the best it can be, even in adverse situations. In addition, I wrote a book about my true-life struggle with dysthymia titled *Born Mad,* and I work to create awareness for this disorder. I am speaking with politicians to create a state and national day designated for dysthymia awareness.

One must tread through the rough waters in order to reach the smooth sailing that follows. Life isn't always a walk in the park, but it shouldn't be a continuous battle either. Don't give up. Keep seeking and be willing to do whatever it takes to find peace and happiness.

Medication was the key for me. Now that I have become stabilized on the proper medications, the other skills and tools I have learned along the way are much more readily maintained and utilized.

Mild depression should not be brushed off and ignored, as it can very quickly and easily turn into major depression.

Dysthymic disorder almost killed me. I write about my struggles with dysthymia to help others who have been diagnosed and those who have not and are wondering what is wrong with them.

For me, dysthymia means frequently making poor decisions, and feeling guilty over things that most wouldn't think about twice. Dysthymia means being moody, frequently mad, sometimes all day, a week or even longer. Dysthymia means getting easily frustrated when things don't go as planned and then not knowing how to solve the problem. For me, taking the proper medication was the key to pulling my life together. I tried various non-pharmaceutical methods of treatment and some had temporary benefits. But after I began taking medication, all those other methods could be utilized more fully. Do I still have bad days and make "not the best" decisions? Yes, but not as often as I used to. Most of my anger has gone away, and I am now able to solve problems better than I have in my entire life.

Robyn Wheeler
Texas, USA
Author of *Born Mad* (2011) and
***104 Ways to Starve Your Anger & Feed Your Soul* (2013)**

The Future Looks Bright
for the First Time

I was first diagnosed with dysthymia by my family doctor when I was 57. We had talked from time to time about my depression (only because it seemed to be getting worse than usual), but I always balked at her recommendation to see a therapist or try medication.

You see, I had dysthymia for 40 years before I learned what it was, so it was deeply entrenched in my mind that it was just who I was and nothing could be done about it. The day I read of her diagnosis, I immediately looked it up in Wikipedia. I almost fell off my chair when I read the symptoms, which matched how I'd been feeling for 40 years.

Now, I can see many of the symptoms actually occurred in my early childhood. It was such a tremendous relief to know that after all these years it was not my fault and I could now put a name to it.

I'm currently taking medication and seeing a therapist. Progress is very slow and often incredibly frustrating. I have to keep reminding myself that all this has been a part of my life for so very long, that it's not going to go away quickly.

I'm so uplifted by reading about others with the same struggles because no one has understood me all this time.

The future looks bright for the first time, though I often have to fight to see it. Many times I feel like I've taken two steps forward and one step backward.

It's very hard to be patient with myself because now that I know what is going on, I want to be done with it.

When I remind myself that it's one day at a time, I have better focus and more patience with myself. We can all get through this!

K. Burke
Baltimore, Maryland, USA

The Trigger to Anger

I feel my anger is triggered when my laid-out plans are unsettled, whether it's a plan to do my best that is suddenly derailed by unseen outside influences or just bad luck. My anger arises when I feel robbed of the success I was striving for.

My ego kicks in, to defend the overwhelming sense of injustice causing me to strike back at whatever or whoever has insulted or stopped my goals from succeeding.

Instead of allowing for other's mistakes, my anger at a perception of their bad judgement takes over me.

The result afterward is a feeling of embarrassment and shame for allowing my negative emotions to get the better of me. There is also a short-lived euphoria from releasing the anger that is usually overcome by the shameful feelings for hurting someone's feelings and lashing out like an insane person. Sometimes the shame is not there if the person I perceived to be causing me a problem is really to blame.

The perception of a wrongful act against me causes me uncomfortable angry feelings. The natural reaction for me is to defend myself or to try to make things "feel right" by expressing the anger. I then feel vindication that what made me angry has been correctly addressed and I can return to feeling normal. In the moments of an anger event, I have to weigh in on whether to respond at all, how to respond, or feeling more anger unrequited from not responding. I do not try to use anger to ruin someone, or to provoke another to become angry or sad. I do it to relieve an intense emotion I'm not comfortable having to deal with.

D. Engelhardt
Minden, Nevada, USA

Believe in Yourself

I was first diagnosed with dysthymia in 2006. Initially what I thought was just stress related from working in the human services field was much more. I was feeling constant anxiety and pessimism and was easily discouraged. It was not getting better on its own, and that is when I sought help.

As a psychology major, I remember learning about dysthymia but did not think that I could very well have it. I have been in counseling off and on since 2000. I would attend some counseling sessions, start to feel better and not feel the need to continue unless I started having problems again. The first time I saw a psychologist was on campus in my sophomore year of college, mainly due to personal problems and social anxiety. My nephew, who was just 3, had moved out unexpectedly over the summer with his mother. I was very close to him, as he had been living with my mother, father, brother, sister-in-law, and me. This situation did not help the down times I was experiencing. In 2005, a psychologist I was seeing told me that I had traits of dysthymia, but I do not remember officially being diagnosed with it until a year later.

Medications have been a challenge throughout my diagnosis, and I have certainly had my share of them. My experience has involved side effects such as sweating, irritability, anxiety, crying spells and sleeping difficulty. Unfortunately, there is no magic pill, nor a cure for this mood disorder. It is one that we must learn to live and cope with. Medication along with therapy is the key to self-improvement.

But more so, it is about simply having a handle on understanding dysthymia. However, it takes a while until you find what works best for you.

Sometimes I think I have had dysthymia my entire life. I remember as a kid reminiscing about things having gone wrong in the past at a time when things were going all right and just making myself all upset. I would start crying and sometimes not understand what made me upset in the first place. What would make me think of things to make me unhappy?

I had friends when I was younger, but junior high and high school proved difficult. I considered myself unique and an outcast from my peers. My interests were different, and conversations were not easy to strike up. When I would speak, it always seemed like something came out wrong. I was made fun of, which did not help matters. Therefore, I refrained from enjoying a lot of activities by my own volition. Today I have many regrets, as I wish I could have been a more outgoing person than such an introvert. I was Most Shyest in my senior yearbook. I suppose I earned it.

You will find that there are many people who do not understand dysthymia. Although a mild depression, it has days where it pulls one down. If left untreated, it could lead to major depression. People could be very quick to judge because they see you working, attending school, going to the movies, just performing daily activities. But they only see the outside, the mask that we all wear. They don't feel the hurt or have to bear the daily struggles that we do. Maybe those individuals are wrapped up in their own problems that make them so quick to judge others without really taking the initiative to understand. While it can be no easy task to educate friends and loved ones on dysthymia, fear not. It can be done.

In 2009, I lost my older brother, my only sibling, unexpectedly. It was the Wednesday before Easter. Then in

2011, my father died unexpectedly. I never imagined my family would be cut in half by the time I was 31. As sensitive as I was when I was younger, and as spontaneous as a crying spell could be for me in public, I just couldn't bring myself to cry following their deaths. I felt very bad, of course, and deeply saddened.

To this day not a single day goes by that I do not think about either of them. While these experiences caused a lot of difficulties for me, they did help me to become a stronger person. However, I must admit that there are times when the going gets so tough that I ask my brother and father to take me with them, to not let me suffer anymore. I know this is not a good way to think and fortunately, I never did nor do I have a plan to end my life. They obviously see me as a stronger person than I do and evidently I am still here for a reason. In life, we will get knocked down, often too many times to count. But we have to be able to get back up and keep going. We are nowhere near the finish line yet.

We can't give in to dysthymia. If we do, it will eat us alive. Instead of looking at it as a weakness, we could make dysthymia a strength. As I stated earlier, one needs to have a handle on this condition. That means taking in all of the necessary knowledge that you can. I found it particularly helpful reading books about dysthymia and joining groups on Facebook where I could talk to others going through the same as me. The Internet is a valuable tool as well.

Today, although much more improved, I can't say that I'm 100%. I never will be and have already accepted that. I take an anti-anxiety medication and an antidepressant. I keep in regular contact with my counselor and I know he is available if I need him. I am married now for nearly five years. I have the support of my family, a stable job and home.

Most importantly above all else is to count your blessings. In the end they are what really matter. Don't forget to take care of and believe in yourself too.

D. Brennan
Pennsylvania, USA

Get Help Sooner Rather than Later

My journey with dysthymia started about 30 years ago. I'm sure I had a predisposition to this disorder, but my symptoms did not manifest until I got married at 26. I know this is what "pulled the trigger," so to speak.

Here is my story.

I grew up in a basically "normal" family with two siblings. I was a fairly happy kid, teenager and young adult.

I met my husband a few years after college at 24. Within a year of getting married, I started to have what I would call anxiety. I did not have panic attacks or severe anxiety, just a general feeling of uneasiness and "not feeling like myself anymore." I did not feel sad or depressed but learned that anxiety is a part of depression.

I knew this was not normal, and it was very scary because I didn't know what was happening to me. Lying in bed one night, I told my husband. He was baffled and didn't really understand what I meant.

I went to a psychiatrist and he put me on the tri-cyclic anti-depressants (all they had back then). I'm not really sure they did much good, but I took them for about a year.

I wanted so badly for everything to be okay that when the New Year started, I made a resolution (of sorts) that the problem was just gone. I went off the medication and stopped seeing the doctor. This happened over and over throughout the years and I would try all kinds of other things to get better and "will myself that everything was okay." You can't wish dysthymia away. It used to be called "low grade" depression, but don't be fooled. Over time, it will wear you down and can easily turn into major depression. It is too powerful for even the strongest of people. That is why it is so important to get help sooner rather than later.

Fast-forward 15 years. I still did not feel like myself, but I did not know what to do about it either. I functioned fairly well to the outside world. During this time, my husband and I had two children and I worked part-time in healthcare.

Over the years, I tried so many things, including exercise, being outside in the sunshine, meditation, religion, yoga, tapping, deep breathing, energy healing, healing touch and working with a life coach. Nothing changed.

Just a little about my marriage and work life, as it is important in telling my story.

Looking back, I think I was not ready for the huge commitment of marriage. I think I got married because all my friends were and my husband was "a nice guy."

I had always pictured myself a strong, independent and career-minded woman. My husband and I were opposites, which can work very well for some people. I was a free-spirit, fun loving and laid back. He was a very serious, regimented, "do everything by the book" kind of guy.

Back then, I felt like he had sucked the life and joy out of me and that I had lost myself. Since then, I have divorced him, after 29 years of marriage.

Regarding my career, I often chose to work part-time and even stepped out of the work world for a while. This was a huge mistake, as it sent me into a deeper depression. My children are my priority, but I need to work in order to feel whole and like I am contributing to something outside the home.

So why did I drop out of the one thing I loved the most? About age 44–45, I started to go downhill. The worst thing was the irritability and anger I felt over the smallest of things, especially with my husband and strangers. It was very disturbing, as I had always been very calm and easy-going and could hardly remember a time when I was hostile or angry.

I also started isolating myself in the bedroom more and more, especially from my husband. About this time, I went to my family doctor, asking for an anti-depressant. He put me on a low-dose anti-depressant that I took for the last 10 years. He said I had a "low-grade" depression. I thought that meant it was not a big deal. He made it seem that way, too.

The next few years were very tough. Here were some of my thoughts and feelings:

- Moving into our "dream House," I thought surely this would get better in this beautiful house out in a beautiful country setting. But something was terribly wrong.

- A few weeks before Christmas, knowing things were so wrong and on the verge of tears, I decided to get my hair highlighted to feel better. I remember wanting to tell my hairdresser how bad I felt, but I didn't.

- Life shouldn't be this hard.

- I was feeling so low that the only thing I could do was concentrate on a few ladybugs that had escaped into our house on the inside of the window. Somehow animals, creatures of any kind, calmed me down, as they represented a "life force."

- Many times I was thinking about suicide in an abstract sort of way but did not actively plan anything.

But the absolute worst thing to happen was yet to come. Something I held so dearly for my well-being, livelihood and reason to get up in the morning: Over the last four years I had lost two jobs due to my anger issues. *This was my breaking point!*

I had felt suicidal before, but this was the real deal. I now had no husband and no job, and my kids were almost grown. What was I going to do, and would I ever get well? I truly felt helpless. I had been trying to fight all these years on my own and could not take it anymore. I looked up ways to kill myself and tried to summon the courage to commit suicide, but in the end I could not do it. (I knew of too many botched suicides.)

I knew this time I really needed to reach out for help. I went to an anger management psychologist. He immediately said I needed to see a psychiatrist. I balked, as I thought, *I am already on medication. What more can I do?*

Boy, am I glad I went for help! The psychiatrist I saw was so warm and caring. He immediately said, "The psychologist and I are going to help you."

Somehow, I knew this time it was true and burst into tears. After all these years, I was getting help! He started me on a low dose and worked me up to a therapeutic dose. That did the trick!

After about three weeks on the right dose, all of a sudden the meds kicked in. It was like I went to bed one person and woke up a different person, more like person I knew I should be. The racing thoughts were gone, the irritability was way down and the impulsivity was down too. It was amazing! And to think I could have gotten this kind of help much sooner.

The medication was the key for me. I know I will need meds for the rest of my life, and I am okay with that.

If you suspect you or a family member has depression, seek help! There is no shame in seeing a psychiatrist and taking medication. It is just like any other physical illness— similar to a diabetic without insulin. It is not your fault! Although I am just a few months out from my transformation, I know with the help of my psychiatrist and medication, I am now going to be fine and can start enjoying life again!

Anonymous

Dysthymia Diagnosis: A Revelation

Everyone always called me a sensitive child. I cried when I was praised, slighted, unhappy or delighted. I worried about school, friends and the day ahead.

As I grew older, I would purposely be the different one, the outsider, so that I would not have to try to learn the secret ways of the popular people.

I disdained emotions and wanted to be purely logical. I wanted to find some way to just live my life without all of the drama. But even so, I felt the tangle of emotions.

I studied sciences, intent on understanding what made things and people function. After graduation, I found working in an educational role gave me a focus and purpose that helped me interact well with others. I found a way of behaving meaningfully and gained a lot of satisfaction.

Somehow, miraculously, I married and had a wonderful son, but still the doubts and swings of emotion pulled.

When my father died, I went through a major depression and found that Zoloft and counseling helped immensely. I was 45 years old.

It was then that I was diagnosed with dysthymia.

What a revelation. All the highs, lows, anger and doubt made sense. I made it through the episode and even managed quite well during a later loss of employment in the great 2008 debacle.

I struggle with anger occasionally, but I feel a lot more forgiving of myself and others these days. In my early retirement,

I rediscovered motorcycling and have completed several solo cross-country tours. This satisfies my restless nature.

Looking at my family, I would say my grandmother dealt with dysthymia all her life, as I do. My mother also struggled with this; she left one job in her mid-40s, staying home without talking about her problems for at least six months.

I feel blessed with my family support and understanding and would wish others the same vital foundation. I keep learning and dealing with my tendency to remain aloof.

I haven't taken medication for years, but I lead a satisfying retired life taking painting classes and the solo trips when I feel the need to examine my thoughts more closely.

C. Freeman
Massachusetts, USA

Part 2:

Putting the Pieces Together

Suggestions for a Happier Life

Dysthymic disorder doesn't feel "mild" to those who suffer from it. It is something a person just wants to get rid of and wishes they didn't have. But it is a constant, lifelong condition. However, with counseling, medication, alternative therapies or other types of treatment, one may find a method or methods that help lessen the frequency and intensity of the symptoms. This chapter is about putting the pieces together to allow yourself to feel the best you can and cope effectively with dysthymic disorder.

Notice this chapter is not titled "Suggestions for a *Happy* Life." I use the word *Happier* on purpose. Dysthymics can live happier and experience joy. They may not be as happy as someone who does not suffer from dysthymic disorder, but they can achieve a happier state of mind than previously experienced with untreated dysthymia.

Since my diagnosis in 2010, I've learned to live with and accept my dysthymic condition. I learned to recognize when I'm stressed, when I need to relax and when I need to step back and take a break from what I'm doing.

My suggestions for living a happier life with dysthymic disorder are included in this chapter. These suggestions do not come from a book written by a doctor, nor do they come from a list of "Top 10 Ways to Deal with Dysthymia," as I'm not sure such a list even exists. They are my tried-and-true experiences in dealing with and handling my own mood disorder to improve the quality of my life. They are things I practice daily and have found useful in coping with the ups and downs, and negativity and frustrations of dysthymia.

You may find some suggestions work for you and some don't. You may add different items to your list. Remember, not all people who suffer from dysthymia experience the same frequency or intensity of symptoms or for that matter, the same symptoms at all.

Although dysthymic disorder is not curable, using the following suggestions along with medication, counseling or whatever method of treatment you choose, may help you become a "happier" person.

I've focused on the mental and emotional aspect of coping with dysthymia. I've also separated these items according to the two types of dysthymia: *anxious* and *anergic*. Just because these items are listed in one of the two categories, it doesn't mean the suggestions cannot be used for both types of dysthymia. Pick the ones you feel you want to work on first or that will help you the most. Start with one and then work on another.

Hopefully, by now, if you suffer from dysthymia, you have an idea of which category you fall into.

For Those with Anxious Dysthymic Disorder

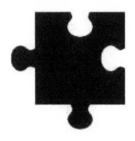

Argue with Yourself

This may not sound like it would be a good thing, because, after all, who likes arguing? But debating one's thoughts can be of benefit to those whose first thought is usually negative and/or self-defeating.

For example, when my first thought is "I'm not smart enough" or "I'm stupid and dumb," I follow that thought with *Okay, so I'm not Bill Gates, but most people aren't. I have a Bachelor of Science degree; I'm certified in anger and stress management and I am a published author. I'm far from dumb. I have all the intelligence I need to succeed at the things I want to succeed at.*

For someone with constant degrading thoughts about oneself, positive thinking and "talking yourself out of it" can make a tremendous difference.

When I am able to talk myself out of my first thought by contradicting it with a second, I am more likely to move on, abandon the "pity party" and accept myself for who I am. Acceptance of oneself is often extremely difficult, if not impossible, for someone living with dysthymia. However, it is a key ingredient in a happier and better quality of life for anyone with a mood disorder.

For more examples of come-backs to specific negative thoughts, see the Helpful Worksheets section in the back.

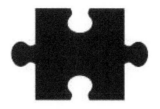

Enough Is Enough:
Reduce Stress

Know your limits, when you've had enough of something. If you have too many things going on, too many commitments, you'll be stressed and more likely to get mad or irritated with yourself. Know at what point you need to stop doing a certain task. Are your signals swearing, yelling, crying, etc.? When your stress point shows its ugly head, quit, take a break, meditate, do something to cool off and calm down. Not all stress is bad; but when stress is dictating your behavior, taking a toll on your health or relationships, it's time to modify your lifestyle.

Don't be afraid to say no. If you already have a full plate and "too many irons in the fire," don't agree to do something else when you are asked. Just say no. You don't have to give an explanation; but if you feel you must, say, "I have a lot of obligations already and don't wish to become rushed, worried or commit to something I probably don't have time to do." Personally, every few months I like to evaluate my activities and commitments and purge a few items if necessary. It is very important for those with either type of dysthymia to include some down time in their day—every day. Take time to enjoy a movie, read a good book, go for a walk in an arboretum or park. Choose what you enjoy and do it. For example, I enjoy listening to music, putting together jigsaw puzzles and playing a few, select games on my phone. Pick what you enjoy and make time every day to do at least one of those things. Avoid allowing yourself to be overcommitted. No one can be happy when they don't have any time for themselves and are always on the run.

Avoid Criticizing and Name-Calling

Many of us with dysthymic disorder have a tendency to criticize ourselves and others. Excessive criticism is unhealthy for you and those around you. Instead of pointing out the wrong things people do, try complimenting yourself and others on something they did right. I find I am happier and can take better control of my disorder if I avoid using terms like "jerk," "idiot," or other derogatory terms. No one likes to be called names, and most namecallers don't feel good about themselves when they use non-specific terms.

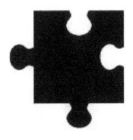

Avoid Exaggerating or Catastrophizing

Many people with dysthymia naturally exaggerate. It's not that we like to embellish, it just seems to be something we learned as children, or part of the intense anxiety that may accompany dysthymic disorder. Sometimes it is difficult not to exaggerate, especially when recalling an event that just recently happened in your life. I've found the anxiety that accompanies my dysthymia is not as great if I force myself to bring things down to reality. That means avoiding saying things like:

- It ruined my life *or* My life is ruined.
- My day was horrible, horrific, disastrous, etc.
- I'm so stupid, ugly, fat etc.
- I can't do anything right.
- I just screw up all the time.
- I hate my life.

Keep the thoughts in your head real. Avoid using words such as always, never and other all-or-nothing terms.

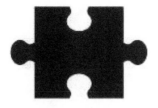

Detach from the Problems
of Others

This one took me a long time to learn. I was in my 40s before I realized being co-dependent was not good for me. And I was bringing it all on myself. Whether a friend, family member of coworker comes to you with a problem, don't get sucked in. Avoid getting upset because they are upset or worrying about their problem because they are worried. You have your own circumstances and adversities to deal with; don't pile on unnecessary baggage by getting involved in someone else's life or circumstances.

This doesn't mean you can't lend an ear when someone comes to you for advice, but avoid getting involved or taking on something that will cause more stress in your life.

Remember the saying: *There are three kinds of business—yours, other peoples and God's.* You are only entitled to yours.

Let other people deal with their business so you can more effectively deal with yours.

Find Daily Enjoyment

Since those who suffer with anxious dysthymia tend not to experience joy as often as others, it is important for us to find things we like to do and do them daily or at least weekly. I like to listen to music, work jigsaw puzzles, color, make crafts, go to the movies, go out to eat and read. The list goes on. Find time every day to do something that will put a smile on your face and make you happy. You decide what that is. Don't let anyone else decide for you. Don't be afraid to try something new. If someone asks you to go to karaoke and you've never been before, go, what have you got to lose? You might like it. How about zip-lining, yoga or dancing? Find something fun, just for you.

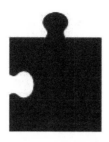

Utilize Self-Help Information

Getting and using self-help information is easily done in today's day and age. Whether you prefer the Internet, books, CDs, audiotapes or some other medium, obtaining self-help information is easy and affordable.

Books have been written by great authors on just about any topic you can think of. Authors such as Dr. Wayne Dyer, Caroline Myss, Louise Hay, Dale Carnagie, Zig Zigler, Cheryl Richardson, Dr. Phil McGraw and Joel Osteen have numerous self-help items available for purchase. And many have free weekly or monthly e-mail newsletters chock full of self-help tips and ideas.

Whether you need help with building self-esteem, controlling anger, engaging in self-care, being more independent, overcoming eating disorders, coping with mental illnesses or conquering your debt, there is a book, CD or Internet video to give you advice.

Make good use of the information available by the experts. Don't just listen or read, but practice what they say in your daily life. Remember, you will not change if you continue to do things the way you've always done them. Change can be difficult for many people; however, change is not only good but necessary for personal growth. Step outside your comfort zone and try something new. You may just find something that changes your whole life and way of thinking for the better.

Some of the best websites for self-help information are www.hayhouse.com, www.thework.com, www.selfgrowth.com, www.successimo.com and www.selfhelpzone.com.

These are just a few. Type in 'self-help websites' and more will pop up in whatever search engine you use.

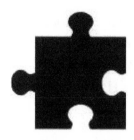

Use Affirmations

I love affirmations. Affirmations usually begin with "I" and then are followed by a positive thought. I began using them after my diagnosis in 2010 and found a large percentage of my dysthymia issues stemmed from a poor outlook on life and negative perceptions of just about everything. I found that saying affirmations after I woke up and before turning in for the night changed my thoughts about myself, life in general and dealing effectively with adversity.

My favorite affirmations are listed below. I did not write these affirmations. I found them online by Dr. Wayne Dyer, Louise Hay and others when I was seeking ways to conquer my anger and improve my quality of life.

- *I do not have any problems, I only* think *I do.*
  —Dr. Wayne Dyer

- *Be better than you used to be.* —Dr. Wayne Dyer

- *I can do all things in Christ who gives me strength.* —Philippians 4:13

- *I am a universal, infinite and divine being capable of anything.* —Dr. Wayne Dyer

- *I am worthy.* —Louise Hay

- *I love myself and only good awaits me at every turn.* —Louise Hay

- *I am getting better and better every day in every way.* —Louise Hay

- *I am worth loving.* —Louise Hay

- *I am willing to learn something new every day.* —Louise Hay

- *I always have a choice.* —Louise Hay

- *I am my own unique self.* —Louise Hay

- *I am willing to change and grow.* —Louise Hay

Below, are sayings I remind myself of on a daily basis or when I face adversity. I say all of them or maybe one or two that fit my particular situation.

- *Don't believe everything you think.* —Dr. Wayne Dyer

- *When you have a problem, there isn't something to do, there is something to know.* —Sylvia Browne

- *Forgiveness is the answer to almost every problem.* —Dr. Wayne Dyer

- *Be the experiencer, not the experience: Say to yourself, "I am the who calls myself a _____ (fill in the blank)."* —Dr. Wayne Dyer

- *There are no coincidences—everything happens for a reason and a purpose.* —Sylvia Browne

- *This too shall pass.* —Ancient Jewish Folklore

- *Progress is impossible if you do things the way you've always done them.* —Dr. Wayne Dyer

- *Today is entirely up to me.* —Dr. Wayne Dyer

- *There are no justified resentments.*
  —Dr. Wayne Dyer
- *The difference between success and failure is perception.* —Dr. Wayne Dyer
- *Avoid making fear-based decisions.*
  —Sylvia Browne
- *All is well in my world.* —Louise Hay
- *Keep your heart free of hate, your mind from worry; live simply, expect little, give much. Fill your life with love, scatter sunshine, forget self and think of others, and do as you would be done by.* —Norman Vincent Peale

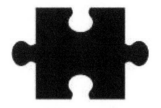

Learn to Laugh

Laughter is truly the best medicine. It is easier to laugh at the funny, lighthearted stuff. It is not so easy to laugh at adversity, but it can make the situation and your soul feel a little bit more lighthearted. If you are faced with a difficult decision and brood over it, get angry and take it too seriously, you'll probably make the wrong decision. Making jokes at yourself and your situation can lighten your mood, allowing for more positive thoughts to override the negative thoughts.

For instance, I write for a newspaper for a living, and just recently a man I had spoken to on the phone filed a complaint about me. Over the next week, he contacted my supervisor, demanding I be terminated. He wrote several e-mails stating I do not "make a pimple on an ant's ass of a reporter" and that I was "an overeducated idiot with the liberal establishment." He even posted a blog on his website about what a horrible reporter I was.

I could have gone home, cried, yelled and screamed, and called him names, justifying the name calling because he did it first. I could have stayed angry and resentful for weeks, months or even years.

Instead, I laughed. Not only had he called me hilarious names that I'd never been called before, but I actually felt sorry for him. How can I resent someone who is obviously so miserable and angry?

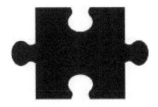

Know Yourself

Knowing your own likes and dislikes, wants and needs and other characteristics about your personality can be very beneficial. Allow the little quirks, traits, and habits to work for you, not against you.

For instance, I know I stress out when I work too much. For most of my life, I've held down more than one job and even volunteered a few places while working two jobs. Now, as I get older, I am slowing down and actually *want* to slow down. I don't want to work two jobs. I'm happier working one, even if it doesn't pay much and is not full time. If I can make ends meet, I'd rather work less, have more time to spend with family and friends, and maybe see a movie once in a while. Work is overrated. If you don't want to be a workaholic, don't. Cut back, for the sake of your mental sanity.

I also don't function well without enough sleep. If I've been up all night or have to wake up extremely early, I'm usually not very talkative, alert or willing to do the things I need to do. I'm grumpy. So, I try to arrange my daily schedule so I don't have to wake up at 4 or 5 a.m. Some people are early morning risers. I'm not one of them. I'm happier if I sleep until at least 8 a.m.

I also don't like large projects or having too many things to think about at the same time. If I have to complete a large project, I try to break it down into smaller, more easily completed tasks. Then, I begin with the smaller things that can be finished more rapidly. I like to get the small tasks out of the way first and then tackle the larger ones. I also don't procrastinate. I won't do well if I wait until the last minute to do anything. I'm always early, whether it is for an appointment, making a phone call or picking up a package. Whatever it is, I'll be early.

If it helps, write down your little quirks; the things you like to do, dislike doing, and just plain don't want to do *ever*. Write down how you like things done. Are you organized, or do you find things more easily when your desk is complete chaos? Take the way you like to do things and make it work for you. If you find a trait or habit you don't like about yourself and it is not working for you, change it. Remember: The definition of insanity is doing the same thing over and over again expecting different results. The only way to get a different, better result is to stop doing things the way you've always done them.

The same mind that created the problem cannot solve the problem. A different way of thinking can and will solve the problem.

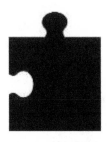

Forgive

Webster's New World College Dictionary defines *forgiveness* as "to give up resentment against or the desire to punish; stop being angry with."

Forgiveness is one of the most important things we can do for ourselves and others, yet it is one of the most difficult things for most people to grant. Many folks have tremendous misconceptions about forgiveness, including:

- He/she should apologize before they receive forgiveness.

- What he/she did was unforgiveable.

- He/she doesn't deserve forgiveness.

- Forgiveness means I've accepted and/or approved of what the other person did.

- Forgiveness means not seeking justice for a wrongdoing.

Forgiveness is not mandatory for life—many people live with their resentments for years and years after the event occurred, and some would rather die with their resentments that let go.

But if a person wishes to live "happy," forgiveness of yourself and others is mandatory. Remember the section of

The Dysthymia Diaries to help those suffering with dysthymia to live a "happier" life. Forgiveness is a gift you give yourself.

The first step is learning to forgive yourself. Easier said than done, right? Those with dysthymia tend to beat themselves up over and over again for making a small, simple mistake. We believe we should be perfect. Next time you find yourself berating yourself, remind yourself that no one on this planet is perfect and no one will ever be perfect. We all make mistakes. We all do things we regret afterward. The trick is to remind yourself that you are doing the best you can, given your particular knowledge, circumstances and skills. No one likes screwing up. But screwing up is a fact of life. It just is. Don't try to fight or resist what is.

I love the saying, "Holding on to resentment is like swallowing poison and expecting the other person to die." Would you physically swallow poison and hope the other person dies? Probably not. So why are you doing it mentally and emotionally?

Forgiveness cannot be based on whether someone deserves it, nor can it be based on an apology. Example: Adam Lanza shot and killed more than 26 children in the Newtown, Connecticut, massacre and then died at the hands of law enforcement. If the parents of those murdered children are waiting for an apology, they will never get it. They have a choice—forgive and move on, living life to the fullest extent, or hold on to resentment forever and be unhappy. All wrongdoings, whether rape, murder, theft, betrayal or otherwise, can be forgiven if you set your mind to it. Besides, where would you draw the line for those you forgive and those you do not forgive? Will you forgive a person who commits a misdemeanor but not a felony? Will you forgive a person without freckles but not those with freckles? I am exaggerating, but do you get my point?

In forgiveness, try this simple step. Imagine you are in their shoes. See things from their perspective. Can you feel empathy for that person? Is it possible they were going through tough times and lashed out at you or made a rash decision?

Also, think of this. If you are a dysthymic who has difficulty making decisions, controlling anger or expressing your wants, needs and feelings, can you see how others may have the same difficulties? Maybe the person who wronged you suffered from a more devastating disorder than yours. Maybe they are struggling with bipolar disorder, obsessive/compulsive disorder, schizophrenia or a personality disorder.

Forgiveness may not come right away, and it certainly doesn't mean you can't seek justice for someone who committed an illegal act against you. You can seek justice and forgive too.

Forgiveness is up to you. You can forgive or not. No one can make you forgive. But you have to forgive if you wish to be happy, live in the present moment and enjoy what's left of the time you have here on earth.

For Those with Anergic Dysthymic Disorder

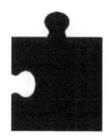

Consider Light Therapy

I have never tried light therapy, but Michael C. Thase, M.D., and Susan S. Lang, authors of *Beating the Blues: New Approaches to Overcoming Dysthymia and Chronic Mild Depression,* wrote, "Exposure to bright light is widely accepted as an effective treatment for seasonal affective disorder. It also is increasingly being considered for the treatment of non-seasonal depression." They also wrote, "Using light therapy with medication and psychotherapy for dysthymia may be synergistic—that is, the effect of them together is greater than just adding the effects of the two of them together; they enhance each other. It also works much quicker (a week vs. several months) and has far fewer side effects than medications."

I put this option in the anergic list because it may increase a person's energy and therefore desire to go out and be proactive in life. This option could also help for those living in a geographic area without a lot of sun or during winter months when the sun sets early in the day. Light units may be purchased and used at home while a person is exercising or watching TV. Light therapy may be better used in the morning or at night, depending on your sleep habits, hormonal changes, etc. Ask your doctor to help you decide what kind of unit to purchase as well as when and how often you should use it.

Light therapy might be worth a try, especially if you don't want to take medication or deal with the side effects of medication.

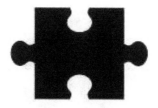

Maintain Social Contact

Avoid sitting around feeling sorry for yourself. Moping can turn a mild situation into a major one fairly quickly. Talk out your situation with a friend, coworker, family member or, if necessary, a radio talk show host. Try surrounding yourself with motivating and inspiring people. I know if I go to dinner with a few motivated women, I come home with ideas turning over in my mind. I can't wait to go home and work on that book, craft project, gardening idea and so on. Dysthymia tends to cause feelings of isolation. Don't get me wrong: Everyone needs "alone time." Some alone time is good for us. But if you are alone too much, dysthymia can become more severe. Social contact with others is necessary for a balanced life and can be beneficial in so many ways. Ask a coworker to grab a cup of coffee or go out for an ice cream, just to talk, even if it's about the latest movie, your job or comment on Facebook or Twitter. Having fun with a friend will give you energy to live your life in a more inspirational way. It will give you energy to do more, be more and accomplish more.

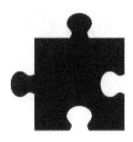

Reward Yourself

Many doctors tell their patients not to diet. Diets don't work because many people feel as though they are denying themselves of the food they love to eat. Diets cause some folks to starve themselves and then binge.

Think of dysthymia the same way. We don't have enough fun or enjoy life as much as others. So reward yourself for nothing in particular. Worked all day and craving a banana split? Then go get one. (Not every day of course.) There are other things you can reward yourself with. Take a long bath or shower, or watch television on your day off. Play a game you like or take the dog for a walk. Don't starve yourself of fun. Try to maintain a "normal" or "average" so you don't binge on something you enjoy. For example, I love Oreos. If I eat one or two Oreos a day, I'm happy. But if I tell myself I can't eat them, go without them for a month and then someone offers me one, I'll go buy a bag and devour it in less than two days. Find a happy medium but reward yourself on a regular basis. You deserve it, and it might just make you a happier person.

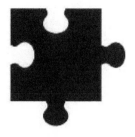

Start Small

I love starting small. If I am faced with a big project that seems overwhelming, I break it down into several parts, starting with the smallest or quickest aspects of the project first and then move on the largest. As a newspaper reporter, I often cover school board meetings. Most of the topics covered require extensive writing; but some, such as moving a board meeting date or approving a field trip, are short and sweet and usually go at the end of the report. So that is where I start, the end. If I write the easy, short stuff first, then I can concentrate on the longer, more laborious items to write about.

All projects can be broken up into parts. Take the time to look over what you need to do and figure out which ones you can do fastest to get them out of the way. Why does this help? Because staring at or struggling with a particular task can wear you down, draining you of energy. If you have relatively low energy to begin with, don't put yourself through the process of being overwhelmed. Start small—then work toward the big stuff. And don't be afraid to take a large part and divide it into "subsections." Create a portion you can deal with, that won't make you feel stressed out or lose interest.

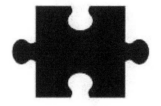

Don't Confuse Your Feelings
with the Truth

Our feelings lie to us. Yes, it's true, how we feel could be nowhere near the truth. And this can trip us up every time if we let it. I once received a letter from a person who said, "I feel like my feelings are foolish and not worth other people's time, and that I am just a weaker human being." This is a perfect example of how feelings can lie to us.

No one's feelings are foolish; all feelings should be expressed and dealt with. You are not a weaker human being, even if you may feel like one. Just because you feel like everyone at work dislikes you, doesn't mean it is true. Just because you feel like you are inferior, doesn't mean it is true. This is when arguing with yourself comes in handy, even a necessity. The arguing-with-yourself tip was discussed under the anxious section, so if you skipped that section, you might want to read it.

Use your logic and common sense to talk yourself out of your negative, unbeneficial feelings. Believing your negative feelings can keep you overwhelmed, unenergetic and less motivated to live your life fully.

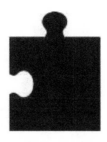

Keep a Log or Journal

Many people are afraid to keep a log or journal but doing so can be of great benefit to most people. If you feel full of energy one day and drained the next, then keeping a journal could uncover some habits or situations that aren't serving you well. Write down what you did, where you went, what you ate, if you exercised, who you argued with, etc., and how you felt throughout the day. If you do this on a day-to-day basis, patterns may appear that could shed light on why you are not energized. Is that nightly cup of coffee keeping you awake? Are you sleeping too much, making you feel groggy all day long? Did you see a movie or have a conversation with a friend that got you motivated? Maybe you argued with a parent or sibling on a regular basis. Does your journal reveal a lot of contact with a person who has a negative effect on your moods? Is there something in your life causing you too much stress or bad feelings?

A journal can help you discover what you need to keep in your life and what you need to eliminate. Don't be afraid to color-coordinate items that show up on a regular basis. Use green for good influences and red for negative ones. Remember, your happiness is of the utmost importance. If something stands out as being of little or no value in your life, consider eliminating it.

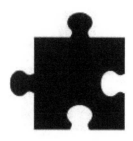

Do Whatever It Takes

We all make excuses once in a while. But the fact is, those who suffer with any kind of disorder need to be determined and willing to do whatever it takes. I've been taking medication for more than five years now. When one medication stops working, I try another. I've taken Zoloft, Cymbalta, Prozac, Welbutrin, Prestiq and currently Lexapro. Do I like taking medications and so many different medications? No, not really. I'd like to stay with one for as long as I can. But medications wear off and may leave a person feeling like they are back to square one. I don't give up, though. I will do whatever it takes. If that means hypnosis, alternative therapy, electric shock—whatever it takes to make me feel happy and peaceful with myself—I am willing to do it.

Never quit trying. Be open-minded. You may think that tapping or meditation is stupid and won't help, but once you try it you may find just the opposite to be true. Try anything. Don't make excuses.

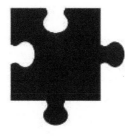

Find a Purpose

Atheists say God doesn't exist and argue with those who believe in God. I say it doesn't matter if God does or doesn't exist. What matters is that you find something to give you a purpose and help you find comfort in this life. If believing in God or a God, makes you feel good about yourself, other people, life in general and the idea that an afterlife follows death, then go ahead and believe.

It doesn't matter whether it is true or not. The only thing that matters is that you find peace, joy and happiness. Then do or use that thing that you found. If believing in angels and unicorns gives you that something you were missing, gives you confidence or the will to improve your life, then post pictures of angels and unicorns all over your house and car and talk to them daily. It doesn't matter if they are real or not. It only matters that they have a positive influence in your life.

Find a purpose or a reason to get out of bed and make the most of your day. You owe it to yourself, your family and others around you. Your life will affect others in the world, whether you personally know them or not.

Ever ask yourself why you have dysthymia? I know why I have it—so I can help others. I wrote my story in *Born Mad*, I taught anger management classes for a brief time and now I have written *The Dysthymia Diaries* to hopefully make an impact on others in the world whom I've never met but who may benefit from reading this book. Some say they want to help other family members deal with dysthymia or other forms of depression. Some say after their diagnosis they want to go out and become the nurse or doctor or therapist they've always dreamed of becoming. You have dysthymia for a reason. But only you can figure out why and where to go or what to do now that you've figured it out.

Find a purpose and a reason for being. Everyone is here for a purpose, including those of us who suffer from mental, emotional and/or physical disorders. In whose life are you making a difference? Do you like to volunteer for animal shelters, nursing homes or child care centers? Do you like to read to others? Play games with seniors at a senior center? Find that purpose, and you will be inspired to be more energetic.

Conclusion

Dealing with Dysthymic disorder is not easy. Life is a challenge for everyone, and suffering from any kind of disorder can make life that much more difficult.

Most individuals who suffer from dysthymic disorder will battle it for their lifetime—every day, every year, into old age. It is not easy, and at times it is downright disgusting, depressing and infuriating. But coping with dysthymia can be a little bit easier to manage by recognizing your symptoms and staying educated.

In 2014, I was diagnosed with type 2 diabetes. I felt depressed, frightened and very angry. But I took a diabetes class and made friends who were going through the same physical and emotional trial I was; and armed with that knowledge, I became less angry, fearful and sad. I know now that I have to take diabetes and dysthymia one day at time.

When my medication wears off and my depression slowly creeps back up, I notice my problem-solving skills diminish. That also means I become more easily frustrated, and then anger sets in: chronic anger that doesn't go away and is directed at everyone in my life.

I use those signs as a gauge for when to call my doctor to discuss other medications or methods that I am willing to try to put my life back in order. Also, keep track of what medications work the best for you. After a year of not being on that medication, you may be able to start taking it again.

Ask your therapist if going back to a previous medication is an option for you.

Knowing yourself, your dysthymia symptoms and being able to act when you need to, will save you a lot of misery. Don't be afraid to ask for help. Remember, keep that journal and take it with you to your doctor appointments for reference.

Use the charts in the Helpful Worksheets section to write down your symptoms and keep track of how they affect your daily moods. If your symptoms are low, you are most likely doing well. But if your symptoms become troublesome for you, you may need to reassess how your therapies are working for you.

Take time every day to assess your dysthymia symptom levels and reevaluate how you are coping with your disorder. If what you are doing is working for you, great. But if not, try something else. Every year, new medications for depression are being created; hopefully, sometime in the near future, dysthymia will be curable. Until then, keep fighting for your life and your happiness. Keep fighting to be the best "you" you can possible be.

I hope *The Dysthymia Diaries* has given you a better insight as to how the disorder can affect individuals, inspired you to find treatments that work for you and left you with some positive thoughts and ideas on how to better cope with the disorder.

Part 3:

Helpful Worksheets

In this section, I've included several forms and worksheets that can be used to help with some of the tips listed in "Suggestions for a Happier Life."

If you already suffer from dysthymia, you can probably benefit from sleep, time, and stress management as well as some form of spiritual and relaxation techniques.

Remember, be willing to try new things and do whatever will help you cope on a day-to-day basis while living with dysthymic disorder. In some of these worksheets you may find help with anger and stress management, scheduling, self-improvement or enjoyable activities.

These worksheets are my creation, but many other forms on the same subjects can be found through various sources, including books, Internet, counseling, etc. I found many similar tools when I was seeking help in balancing and improving my life and coping skills.

Try Metta Meditation

Many people find regular meditation to be beneficial in controlling/coping with anger. The Metta Meditation is easy and incorporates the Buddhist loving-kindness practice with relaxation and visualization techniques.

Here's how to do Metta Meditation:

- Sit comfortably in a peaceful place, breathe deeply and begin to relax.

- Create a sense of acceptance for yourself by saying: *May I be happy, may I be healthy, may I be free from harm, may I be at peace.*

- Visualize a friend or loved one and say: *May (John, Betty, etc.) be happy, may ____ be healthy, may ___ be free of harm, may ____ be at peace.*

- Picture a more distant person like a postman, clerk, or acquaintance and say: *May ___be happy, may ___ be healthy, may ___ be free of harm, may ___ be at peace.*

- Think of someone you may be in conflict with or someone you don't necessarily like or who may not like you and say: *May ___ be happy, may ___ be healthy, may ___ be free of harm, may ___ be at peace.*

- Visualize the world itself and everyone in it and say: *May ___ be happy, may ___ be healthy, may ___ be free of harm, may ___ be at peace.*

Keep a Meditation Journal

Fill in your emotional state after meditating. I've filled in a few for you, but they are by no means an extensive list. Don't be afraid to create your own adjectives below the five I have given you.

	Emotions After Meditating						
	Sun	Mon	Tue	Wed	Thu	Fri	Sat
Calm							
Peaceful							
Relaxed							
Angry							
Frustrated							

Get a Good Night's Sleep

Sleep, exercise and diet are extremely important in managing stress. Sleep is the first and most important of these factors.

- Forty percent of adults admit their quality of work suffers when they are sleepy.

- Sixty-eight percent of adults say that sleepiness interferes with their concentration, and 66 percent say sleepiness makes handling stress on the job more difficult.

- Nearly 24 percent of adults have difficulty getting up for work two or more day per week.

- According to the National Sleep Foundation, approximately 100,000 traffic accidents and 1,500 traffic-related fatalities are caused by a driver who falls asleep at the wheel.

The average adult requires 8 hours of sleep per night, and teenagers require 8.5 to 9.25 hours. If a person does not get enough sleep, the following may occur:

- Anxiety
- Depression
- Irritability
- Suppressed immune system
- Undesirable weight gain
- Increase in making mistakes and having accidents
- Increase in clumsiness and slower reaction times

- Decreased ability to concentrate and understand information
- Sleep disorders: insomnia, snoring, sleep apnea, sleepwalking or restless leg syndrome

Sleep Management Strategies

- Figure out why you aren't getting enough sleep and change your routine. Allow for earlier bedtimes or later wake up times, skip staying up late watching TV or surfing the 'net.
- Create a bedtime ritual. Meditating, taking a warm bath, having cup of tea, reading a book, having a massage and/or journaling all work well right before bedtime.
- Avoid falling asleep in front of the TV.
- Avoid getting stressed about being unable to sleep. Get up, read, meditate or do something else that will make you sleepy. Don't worry; think of positive, relaxing, pleasant things.
- Avoid consuming caffeine after lunchtime.
- Eat a light, healthy dinner with fresh fruits, vegetables and whole grains. Avoid high-fat or over-processed foods. Dinner should be your lightest meal of the day.
- Foods high in tryptophan are good 30 to 60 minutes before bedtime. Consider peanut butter, rice, turkey, milk, dates, figs and yogurt.
- Avoid drink alcohol in the evening.
- Get enough exercise during the day.

Sleep

Good quality sleep and enough sleep definitely affect stress levels.

It is important to do the following:

- Maintain a regular bedtime and wake up time.
- Keep your bedroom dark, cool and free of distractions.
- Have comfortable bedding and pillows.
- Avoid caffeine consumption in the afternoon.
- Discontinue eating two to three hours before bedtime.
- Avoid using a computer or watching TV an hour before bedtime.
- Exercise earlier in the day.

Having trouble sleeping? Drink a cup of warm milk. Milk contains tryptophan and calcium, both of which boost serotonin levels. It also puts you in a good mood. (Do not use this technique if you have milk allergies.)

Manage Your Stress

Stress can be negative or positive. Either way, stress management is necessary for an individual's happiness, health and overall emotional stability. When stress levels become too high, it takes a toll on all areas of a person's life. For each of the items below, think about the past month and indicate how much each item has been a problem for you.

Scale:
1–never, 2–rarely, 3–sometimes, 4–often, 5–always

1. I eat well-balanced, nutritious meals every day.

    1 2 3 4 5

2. I enjoy my work.

    1 2 3 4 5

3. I like myself.

    1 2 3 4 5

4. I exercise regularly.

    1 2 3 4 5

5. I organize and manage my time sufficiently.

    1 2 3 4 5

6. I feel in control, take on new challenges and seek solutions to my problems.

    1 2 3 4 5

7. I speak openly about my feelings.

    1 2 3 4 5

8. I can say "No" easily and without feeling guilty.

    1 2 3 4 5

9. My income is sufficient to pay my bills and allow me to live comfortably.

    1 2 3 4 5

10. I do not drink or smoke in excess.

    1 2 3 4 5

11. I get enough uninterrupted sleep and wake up in the morning feeling refreshed and relaxed.

    1 2 3 4 5

12. I am not overweight for my height and body type.

    1 2 3 4 5

13. I have a good support system of family, friends and recreational activities.

    1 2 3 4 5

14. I am flexible and able to maintain a healthy balance between work, family and recreational activities.

    1 2 3 4 5

15. I consume less than three cups of coffee, tea, sodas or caffeine a day.

    1 2 3 4 5

Add up your scores for all 15 items and use the following scale for an explanation of your scores regarding your stress levels.

1–30: Great.
You are doing a great job maintaining balance in your life. Stress and/or anger management might help you achieve even higher levels of performance.

31–50: Okay.
You are managing stress but could still use some improvement. Stress and/or anger management might help you become more relaxed and at ease with your life.

51–100: Need help.
You most likely need to change some of your behaviors and habits with new and better skills. You most likely could benefit from coaching and/or anger/stress management.

Manage Your Time

Time is a resource, just like your money. Wasted time can be wasted money and create undue stress. Maintaining good time-management habits will make your life easier and less stressful and can change your life. For each item below, indicate how much each has been a source of stress for you in the past month.

Scale:
1–never, 2–rarely, 3–sometimes, 4–often, 5–always

1. I feel overwhelmed by too many tasks and responsibilities and deciding which ones are most important.

     1 2 3 4 5

2. I am very busy and frequently impatient.

     1 2 3 4 5

3. The closer the deadlines, the harder I have to work.

     1 2 3 4 5

4. I have to cope with too many organizational or job-task changes.

     1 2 3 4 5

5. I am drowning in information from mail, faxes, e-mail and the Internet.

     1 2 3 4 5

6. I feel pressure from too many demands from clients/parents/customers/bosses/expectations.

    1 2 3 4 5

7. I dislike turning over responsibility to others.

    1 2 3 4 5

8. I find it difficult to stay agile, flexible and resilient and focus on what is important.

    1 2 3 4 5

9. I worry a lot, and it robs me of time and energy.

    1 2 3 4 5

10. I'm often late for appointments or meetings.

    1 2 3 4 5

11. My *B* and *C* priorities take so much time I rarely get to the *A* priorities.

    1 2 3 4 5

12. I put things off until it is too late.

    1 2 3 4 5

13. I look at projects as a whole rather than breaking them down into smaller sections.

    1 2 3 4 5

14. I do not get enough sleep and do not feel rested in the morning.

    1 2 3 4 5

15. My behavior is opposite of how I truly believe.

     1 2 3 4 5

16. Planning my day-to-day activities is difficult for me.

     1 2 3 4 5

17. I am unable to establish a clear direction and develop personal and career goals.

     1 2 3 4 5

18. I find it difficult to create a healthy work and life balance.

     1 2 3 4 5

Add up your scores for all 18 items and use the following scale for an explanation of your scores regarding your stress levels.

1–30: Great.
You are doing a great job maintaining balance in your life. Time management might help you achieve even higher levels of performance.

31–50: Okay.
You are managing your time to a certain extent, and time management could probably help you to feel more relaxed and at ease with your life.

51–100: Need help.
You most likely need to change some of your behaviors and habits with new and better skills. You most likely could benefit from coaching and time management.

Avoid Exaggerating or Castastrophizing Thoughts

Exaggerated thought	Replace with...
I am stupid.	I have all the intelligence I need.
My life is ruined.	Okay, some things in my life are not the way I want them, but I can change those things with a little effort. I still have a lot of good things going for me.
I screw up all the time. I cannot do anything right.	I don't screw up all the time. In fact, I do more things correctly than I do incorrectly. Everyone makes mistakes. I will learn from my mistakes and get it right the next time around.
That sucks. That's stupid.	Everything and everybody has good points and bad points. Just because something is not what I would do or how I would do it, doesn't mean everyone feels the same way. Some people hate _____, whereas I like _____. And nothing sucks big time! No one likes waiting at the doctor's office, but I can choose to walk out with a treatment for a rash or walk out still needing treatment and suffering. It didn't suck, it's just part of life. (I use this example because I'm not a patient person and don't enjoy waiting for anything, whether at a doctor's office or the grocery store.)

Exaggerated thought	Replace with...
My day was disastrous.	My day wasn't disastrous. Maybe a few things didn't go the way I planned, but most days won't go the way I plan. Most days will require me to be flexible and "go with the flow." (List all the things that went right and wrong. Compare them and you'll probably find only a few things did not go as planned and the majority of your daily events went smoothly. If you misplaced your car keys and were 10 minutes late for work, your day was not disastrous; you were just 10 minutes late for work).
I am a freak, strange, a misfit.	I am unique and special. I may have a few physical, mental or emotional challenges, but who doesn't? We all have to deal with health issues as we get older, and everyone has their own way of doing things. I don't want to be a clone of someone else. I love myself and who I am. Everyone has imperfections. I love my imperfections.

Exaggerated thought	Replace with...
Nothing ever goes right. Why do all the bad things happen to me?	Not all bad things happen to me; they happen to others, too. And many things in my life go smoothly. I cannot expect everything to go smoothly; it won't. Sometimes it is difficult to find a new job, buy a house, deal with large companies about bills, taxes, etc., but most things in life are rarely simple and easy. If I count all the things in my life that have gone right and compare to those that have gone "wrong," the right list will most likely outweigh the "wrong."

Maintain a Relevance Task Chart

Make sure your day is not consumed with "must do's." Make time every day for a balance of tasks. Each day should have must do's, should do's and items that reduce stress. If one day leans too much toward one, use the next day to balance it out. I like to chart things daily on a paper calendar where I can see the entire month. For a more visual display, after writing down your to-do's, highlight your most important to least important tasks using different colors. Too much of one color is not a good balance. I've written some down for you and left room for you to add in your own.

Must do	*Should do*	*Would like to do*	*Reduce stress*
Work	Facebook	Volunteer	Take a bath
Church	Call friend	Go to movies	Do yoga
Visit parent	Clean house	Play computer game	Read a book
Exercise	Do laundry		

Plan Enjoyment or "Me Time"

Spend at least 20 minutes a day doing something you like to do. Chart those activities using the table below, and see if these 20 minutes, over time, will make a difference in your attitudes and emotions. Again, I've left spaces for you to write in your own activities.

	Things I enjoy doing						
	Sun	Mon	Tue	Wed	Thu	Fri	Sat
Reading							
Writing							
Swimming							
Playing video games							

Keep a Daily Journal

Remember, you don't have to change overnight. Look for patterns over days, weeks or months. Try changing one thing, then another. It is "evolution" over time, not a "revolution" overnight. I've created the first journal as an example.

Date	Activities	Who I spoke to	What I ate	Sleep	Exercise	Feelings	Change
2/4	Watched TV	Sister	Donuts	3 hrs	None	De-pressed	Go for a walk
	Took nap	Mother	Soda			Unmoti-vated	Eat healthier foods
		Boyfriend	Ham-burger and fries				Get more sleep

Date	Activities	Who I spoke to	What I ate	Sleep	Exercise	Feelings	Change

Date	Activi-ties	Who I spoke to	What I ate	Sleep	Exercise	Feelings	Change

Date	Activi-ties	Who I spoke to	What I ate	Sleep	Exercise	Feelings	Change

Links and Support

Support Group Information

http://www.bornmad.org/

http://www.mdjunction.com/dysthymia

https://www.facebook.com/DysthymicdisorderInformation/

Hotlines

Suicidal Hotline 1-800-784-2433

Depression Hotline 1-630-482-9696

Teen Suicide Hotline 1-800-784-2433

Find a Psychiatrist

http://www.find-a-psychiatrist.com/

http://www.doctor.webmd.com/

http://www.healthgrades.com/psychiatry-directory

American Psychiatric Association (APA)

http://www.psychiatry.org/

BeliefNet.com

http://www.beliefnet.com/

About Robyn Wheeler

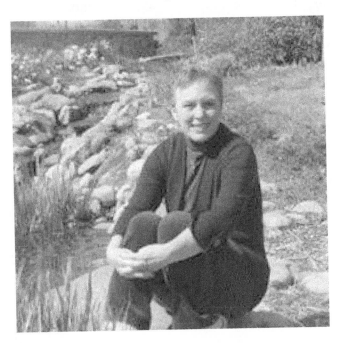

Robyn Wheeler is the author of *Born Mad* and *104 Ways to Starve Your Anger and Feed Your Soul.* She penned *Born Mad* after being diagnosed with dysthymic disorder in 2010 to help others who may unknowingly be suffering from the chronic anger, anxiety and moodiness that may accompany the mood disorder.

Since publication in July 2011, *Born Mad* has received many 5-star ratings on Amazon as well as second place in newbie–nonfiction and women's interest, and honorable mention in cover design and self-help/improvement in the 2012 Royal Dragonfly Book Awards.

Robyn has appeared on numerous television, radio, newspaper, magazine and web outlets.

104 Ways to Starve Your Anger and Feed Your Soul was labeled a "must have" for all school counseling centers by Mabank Independent School District superintendent Dr. Russell Marshall.

Robyn is also the author of *The Creature Teacher's Frog-tastic Funbook* series for children and a contributing writer in Tami Neumann's *Conversations in Care: The Hidden Gems in Dementia & Caregiving.*

Before becoming a writer, newspaper reporter and public speaker, Robyn was the owner of The Creature Teacher, LLC wildlife education service for 15 years.

Robyn is a certified anger and stress management facilitator and graduated from California State Polytechnic University, Pomona, in 1988.

CPSIA information can be obtained
at www.ICGtesting.com
Printed in the USA
BVHW030212090323
659972BV00009B/856